CONTENTS

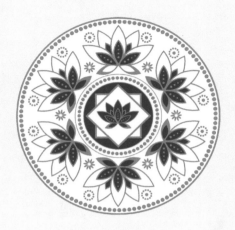

DREAMWORK for GROWTH & HEALING

INTRODUCTION

Almost 20 years ago, my husband died suddenly and unexpectedly, right in front of me; crazed by grief, I left the United States to live in Central America. Shortly thereafter, I remarried, and within a year, I lost a son just 12 days before his due date. Within the next year, I watched my mother die slowly and painfully from colon cancer. In a brief, three-year period, I lost a spouse, a child, and a parent. As I reeled from these tragic events, my oldest son slid into the abyss of addiction and entered rehab. At this point, I figured the worst had to be behind me. Then, seven years ago, I was diagnosed with cancer, received a grueling treatment, and survived.

These traumas could have completely undone me. I could have understandably slid into chronic depression, addiction, or worse. However, during and after these traumatic events, I had the good fortune to be able to consult with my dreams both on my own and with the help of other dreamworkers. My dream imagery showed me resources that I never imagined I had, including hope beyond hope, purpose and strength, and loving support in symbolic guises. As each new trauma rocked me to my core, my dreams compensated by showing me new perspectives and how to find meaning in it all.

From my ability to make meaning out of suffering, and the growth it provided, I discovered my passion and committed to healing myself and facilitating others' healing processes through dreamwork. I can honestly say that my healing and this process of meaning-making occurred as a result of listening to and integrating the soulful guidance from my dreams. I continue to experience greater meaning through bringing what is unconscious into the light of consciousness.

Over the coming weeks and months, I hope that this guided journal will serve you as a tool toward growth, healing, and meaning-making. Ideally, the tools you will learn here will become a resource for you for the rest of your life and one that you will share with others.

What is dreamwork?

Theories on dreams and their meanings have been recorded throughout time by Romans, Egyptians, Hebrew, Chinese, and many others. The ancients believed that the dream was a gift from the gods to direct humans in their lives; they considered dreams to be the medicine of the soul. Five thousand years ago, one would have found Asklepian dream healing centers scattered throughout Greek, Egyptian, and later, Roman cultures. Attendees of these sanctuaries believed healing occurred through the worship of Asklepios and was the direct result of dreaming. People used dream incubation (engaging the dreamer in an active role in communication with the unconscious with the help of a guide or priest) intentionally for healing and guidance on specific issues.

Later on, the famous psychoanalyst Carl Jung defined the dream as "a spontaneous self portrayal, in symbolic form, of the actual situation in the unconscious." Jung regarded dreams as a creative process that situates the dream as a reflection of what is happening in the unconscious. Jung believed that some dream images derive from a collective unconscious rather than solely from the dreamer's personal experiences. The collective unconscious constitutes all aspects of the psyche fundamental to the human condition, characteristics that belong to us by nature. The collective unconscious holds the inherited experiential record of the human species in the form of archetypes.

Jung observed that the images that arise in people's dreams often correspond precisely to the symbols and images that appeared in ancient myths, art, and religion, from times and places that the dreamer could not possibly have known. He called these images archetypes. These images bind us together, and they come from a place where all human potential originates.

In this journal, we will entertain the idea that dreams speak to us in this forgotten language of metaphors, symbols, images, and archetypes. Take the archetype of "the Good Mother," for example. Whether or not we had one ourselves, we share a common understanding that this archetypal good mother exists. We probably have an image that comes to mind as to how she looks. This is an image of an archetype. We dream in archetypal imagery; only the meaning in our dream images is particular to the dreamer. These images and events are not literal but have an archetypal resonance. The hidden symbolism and messages of these dreams are also unique to the dreamer.

All of psychic life rises from these collective unconscious depths, and this is why we spend one-third of our lives asleep so that we can reconnect with our energizing psychic roots. This reconnect restores and balances our conscious mind, supplying us with whatever is missing in waking consciousness. The dream realm is a wondrous universe, full of unseen energies, forms of intelligence, and distinct personalities. It is a much larger realm than most of us realize, one with a complete life of its own that runs alongside our waking life. The dream realm is the secret source of much of our thoughts, feelings, and behavior. Our dream life creates patterns through which individual strands or tendencies become visible. If you watch this meandering design over a period of time, you can observe a sort of regulating or directing trend at work, creating a slow, imperceptible process of psychic growth. With focused attention, one gains insights, perceptions, and even a deeper understanding of oneself – opening a path for a new way forward.

Dreamwork is a process of making meaning out of a world that can sometimes seem cold, random, and impersonal. Engaging with your own symbols and imagery assists you in discovering the messages hidden within. You will be helped and guided by your dream imagery. You will come to trust and value the archetypal nature of these images. Once you allow them equal status with the imagery in your waking consciousness, they will guide you to a deeper understanding of yourself and lead you to a place of healing, love, and creativity. Here, you can integrate these messages into your daily life in a powerful way.

Gaining access to your personal dream realm and its symbolism is an invaluable skill; therefore, I will guide and encourage you every step of the way. Sometimes the issues that the dream realm helps us integrate into our waking lives were relegated to the unconscious during difficult times in our past. In all of my years of practice and counseling (which included many severe cases of trauma), I have come to believe that there is no such thing as a "bad dream."

What may appear as a nightmare or a bad dream is simply material that urgently requires our attention and integration. In the following pages, you will learn to host, attend to, understand, and integrate your dreams in ways that will expand your understanding of your own inner resources and guide you to make meaning of your nightly dreaming adventures.

You will learn step-by-step how to benefit from interacting with your dreams. We are souls with unlimited potential, and you will learn how dreams help us realize this and will access the skills to express this power of creation in our waking world.

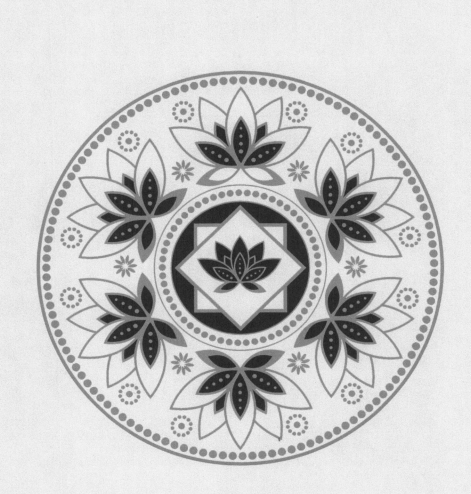

DREAMWORK for GROWTH & HEALING

DREAMWORK for GROWTH & HEALING

STEP ONE

Inviting and Hosting Your Dreams

Remember, dreamwork is a relationship-building process. You are both honing a skill and fostering a relationship. Be patient and encouraging toward yourself. Encouragement for the dream realms simply looks like having your attention on it. Don't disregard anything. Write down everything you dream. Record it. Make a drawing. Write a poem. More will come. As you will see, there are many ways to encourage our dreams. Be gentle with yourself and your dream imagery. Approach this process with the same elements you would bring to any successful relationship: gentleness, kindness, acceptance, trust, and patience. The dream realm will respond to your attention, but the process may take some time to unfold – especially if you are not already an active dreamer and your relationship with your dreams lacks vitality. We all dream. Every night. All of us: man, woman, and child, no matter where we are on Earth or in what circumstances we live. Won't it be incredible when we can begin to make something out of an activity we spend so much of our lives doing?

Here are a few tips to help with dream recall. Find the one that works for you or try them all:

1. To begin with, try to wake as slowly as possible. An alarm clock shatters the hypnagogic state, which is those moments between sleep and wakefulness when our ability to recall dreams is strongest. If possible, when you first wake up, do not jump up or turn your attention to anything. Even if you do not think you can remember a dream, take just a minute to see if there are any feelings or images you can describe. Following this simple step may cause an entire dream to come flooding back.

2. Before sleep, set up a habit of incubating a desire - starting with the desire to have a dream and remember it. Softly or silently speak this desire to yourself as the last thing before you fall asleep. Aim to "feel" the desire

and stay with it for a few moments as the last thing before you sleep. You can get particular about this. For example, you can state, "I'd like to have a dream about (a question or situation), and I want to remember my dream. Spend a minute or two thinking about and feeling into the situation or question you want to dream about just before you doze off.

3. At the beginning, it is essential to establish a relationship with your dreams; therefore, never disregard anything that you recall upon waking, even if it is only one image, a sound, or even a color. Write everything down as a way of establishing a dialogue. Because dream images often make no sense, you may want to dismiss them as weird or meaningless. However, dreams can be quite coherent once we take the time to learn their language. Dreams are not literal but speak a perfect communication composed of symbols specific to the dreamer. This is not meant to confuse us but is the native language of dreams.

4. Don't wait to write down or record a dream thinking you'll remember it later – you probably won't. Write everything down immediately upon waking – even if you wake in the middle of the night. Some people use a lighted pen, in which case they can stay put, which is best. If you worry about disturbing anyone you share your room or bed with, it's best to leave the room quietly with your journal for extensive writing. I sometimes sneak to the bathroom to voice record a dream using my phone.

5. You can also try making sketches of visual memories of a dream to stimulate the arising of more details in your memory.

6. Set up multiple slow, gentle alarms throughout the night. As the brain awakens, it starts to turn on processes needed for long-term storage. Studies show that we remember dreams much more vividly when we awaken directly from the dream. You can do this by setting your alarm to wake you after roughly 4.5 hours of sleep. Use a gentle tone that builds if

you can. With luck, this will wake you during the first chunky phase of REM sleep, and you'll have immediate dream recall.

7. Spraying a natural lavender scent on one's pillow can aid dream recall for some people. Eating foods high in tryptophans a couple of hours before sleep may help others. Dream research shows that vitamin B6 may enhance dreaming; however, it should only be used for short periods (3-7 days to kickstart your dreaming) at a relatively low dose (100-500 mg) as the body doesn't really need it. This protocol seems to work best taken two hours before bed. The supplement 5HTP also works for some as the body naturally converts it tryptophan before it becomes serotonin. Serotonin levels play an essential role in regulating the body's sleep/wake cycle. If you are interested in taking supplements to boost your dream life to the next level, you can also research specially designed dreaming supplements online, including Huperzine-A, DHEA, choline, and mugwort.

8. If you have repetitive dreams or nightmares that have stuck with you over a period of time, please write those dreams down as well; you will most certainly want to take a look at those later. When journaling your dreams, use as much detail as possible. Don't worry about writing style, punctuation, or grammar – just free write – get it down on paper. Write the dream in first-person and be sure it's in present tense. For example, instead of writing "I was standing in a field," write "I AM standing in a field." The idea is to recreate the dream. You can then go back and underline unusual characters, symbols, scenes, plots, themes, or emotions.

"Archetypes and Images."

On this page, list any archetypal images you notice in your dreams. These are all the images that have a shared cultural meaning and significance or that pique your curiosity. If you list a person you know, include their name. We will come back to this practice in a later section, but for now, just list them in one column.

For example:

The Mother

Water

Home

The Door

The Monster

The Friend

The Sexy Lady

Remove all personal meaning for this exercise (we'll get to that in a later lesson) and just think about whether the images have commonly held significance across cultures, religions, locations, myths, and fairytales, etc. Remember, the dream realm responds to our attention, and that honoring the unity of the two worlds makes us whole. When we are just getting started, no snippet of a dream is too small or unimportant. No matter what happens, write everything down along with the date. Don't get discouraged. Keep trying the tips mentioned above alone or in combination, and eventually, you will have just the dream you are meant to have.

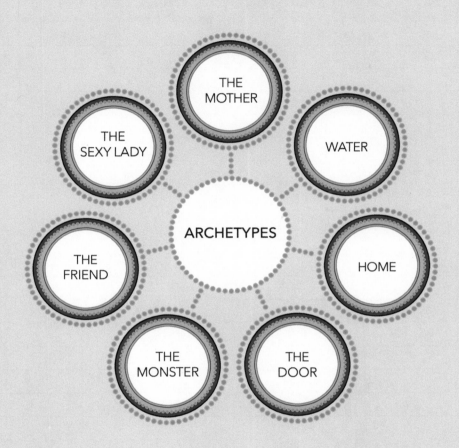

THE
MOTHER

WATER

THE
SEXY LADY

ARCHETYPES

HOME

THE
FRIEND

THE
MONSTER

THE
DOOR

THE DREAM

Title_____

Write down your dream immediately upon waking and give it a title.

Date _____

Day of Week _____

Time to Bed _____

Time Awake _____

☐ Incubated

or

☐ Spontaneous

Mood _____

Develop a bedtime routine. Was the dream incubated or spontaneous? Write down your mood.

_____
_____
_____
_____
_____
_____
_____
_____
_____
_____
_____
_____
_____
_____
_____
_____
_____
_____
_____
_____
_____
_____
_____
_____
_____
_____
_____
_____
_____
_____
_____
_____
_____
_____
_____
_____

ARCHETYPES & IMAGES

On these pages you will list any images that stand out from your dream.

DREAM SKETCH

*Try making sketches of visual memories of the dream
in order to stimulate more details to memory.*

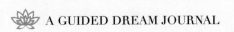

Return to this page after step four.

THE MEANING

*For this step include any understanding you have gained
as a result of examing your associations.*

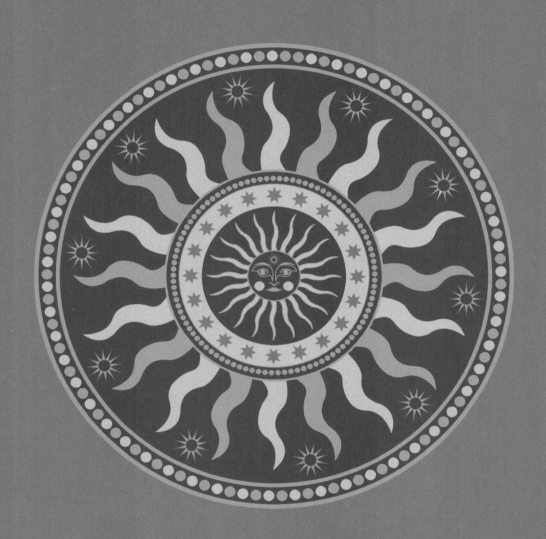

DREAMWORK for GROWTH & HEALING

STEP TWO

Dream Incubation: Dreaming with Intention

We can think of dream incubation as intentional dreaming. Many artistic, conceptual, and concrete creations and innovations have been born out of dream incubation, with varying degrees of intent. Einstein had a dream as a teenager that influenced his theory of relativity, and Nikola Tesla dreamt of the wireless transmission of electrical energy. We also owe penicillin, insulin, and the invention of the computer to dreams.

Dream incubation is an acknowledgment of the two-way relationship between our waking life and our dream life – these worlds are related, and communication is possible between them. Using dream incubation, we can learn to focus on a particular topic while we dream. One of the most important aspects of dream incubation is setting an intention to communicate with your dreams. You must deeply feel the intention-setting process in both your emotional state and your body. The more intentionally you set your incubation, the more likely you will receive a dream in response.

Think of dreams as moments of freedom that allow you to rebuild your emotional and intellectual strength. Approach the dream realm with certainty, knowing that your dreams will help you resolve problems and bring you moments of joy during the night. Your motivation and expectations will create new beliefs.

Before you go to sleep, do some self-inquiry to decide what you would like to be the focus of your dreams. For example, if you are trying to decide between two opportunities, really sense into what it would feel like to be in each scenario. Mentally and physically fill in as many details as you can. Then, before formulating your question about which opportunity is best, set the intention for insight to come to you and let that desire fill your being – what would it feel like to know with 100% certainty that you're making the right choice? Some people find that it helps to write their intention or question down in their dream journal and keep it by the bed while they sleep.

As you fall asleep, recite your intention in your mind until you can really feel it in your body. You might start with a phrase like, "Tonight, I will remember my dreams with ease," or, "Tonight, I will become more aware of my dreams," or perhaps, "Tonight, I want to dream about…"

Patience is vital when incubating a dream. It may take a few days for a dream to come in response to the question or intention you set – the reflection is not always immediate. Other times, it may happen overnight. Either way, know that the reflection is coming, and be prepared and open to receive it when it arrives. I recommend writing down every dream you remember for at least two weeks after a dream incubation. If you don't get a dream in response after a couple of weeks, do the dream incubation several nights in a row.

If you still don't receive a dream, consider a gentle supplement like mugwort or use some of the other methods we covered back in Step One ("Inviting and Hosting Your Dreams"). Remember, your dream will more than likely not seem like a direct response to your incubation. Dreams are not literal, and we will need to learn their language. I know it may sound like I'm repeating myself, but that is how important this is: record EVERYTHING.

You might start out remembering one dream per month; then you may remember two per week, and eventually, you may recall more than one dream per night. As results manifest, you will become more confident in the process; with your certainty, the process will become more easeful. Confidence grows with experience.

STEP TWO

Here are a few suggestions to help you invent incubation requests that match your desire and your creativity. Start with the intention: "Tonight, in my dreams…"

For Work:
- …I will learn why I am unhappy at work.
- …I will discover how to communicate my ideas more effectively.

In Relationships:
- …I will liberate my hidden feelings.
- …I will find new ways to express my sensuality.

For Creative Endeavors:
- …I will discover my creative potential.
- …I will remove blockages that hold me back.
- …I will work on different ways to express myself.

For Emotional Healing:
- …I will understand the cause of my pain.
- …I will meet guides who will help me resolve my fears.

For Personal Growth:
- …I will make room for abundance.
- …I will experience more daring attitudes.

Dreams constantly work to help us, but they do so in their own way. We don't control them, but we can make suggestions or requests. Dream incubation is a gentle way to invite the dream realm's cooperation and focus our healing in a specific direction. Your dreams organize an answer by offering imagery from the databank you accumulate during the daytime and from the symbolic imagery held in the collective unconscious. The soul then sorts this information and channels it for our use. The dream environment's honesty reveals our doubts and our certainties, our weaknesses and our strengths, our sorrows, and our joys. In this realm, we can establish the intention to go beyond ourselves – to transform.

For the ordinary dreamer, night adventures can appear to simply be an escape from daily life, but for the intuitive person, dreams can be a source of guidance and inspiration. For psychotherapy patients, dreams act as a mirror, revealing the psychic causes at the source of current problems. For the truth-seeker, dreamtime experiences become journeys to deeper understanding.

Dreams are journeys into the subtle dimensions of awareness. These journeys give us information about our physical, emotional, mental, and spiritual conditions. The intention underlying dream incubation is to encourage dreams that fulfill our most daring and most exalted wishes and to help us capitalize on our unlimited potential as creators of our reality. The experiences dreams bring are rich with lessons and teachings. For this lesson, incubate and record a dream, along with its images, and in step three, we'll add a translation tool to get closer to the wisdom your dreams are sharing.

" *We must learn how to go into the unconscious realm known as dreaming and become receptive to its messages. This process of self-discovery can be accomplished through hosting and attending to our dreams and the personally meaningful images they hold.* "

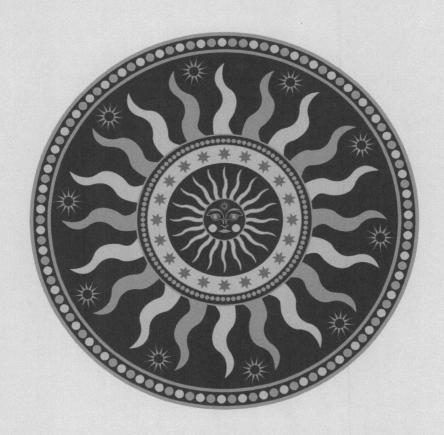

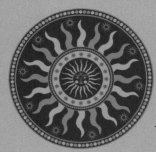

THE DREAM

Title_____

Write down your dream immediately upon waking and give it a title.

What is your intention or question?

_____

Practice: As you prepare for sleep, relax your body, and think about an intention that is extremely important to you. Spend some time sensing into that intention and noticing the feelings that come up and where these emotions arise in your body. Connect to what you are feeling, notice where you sense the intention in your body, and approach your dream incubation with certainty that insight will arise related to this aspect of your life and clarity will be revealed. Focus on the sensations and the part(s) of your body that are most stimulated. Stay connected to this embodied state for about 30 seconds before you go to sleep. In the morning, record any aspect you recall of your dream no matter how small. It's important to recall details of each image and scene, as well as the emotions that are connected to each of those images or scenarios - remember to note how the images made you feel in addition to what you saw or experienced.

Date_____ ☐ Incubated

Day of Week_____ or

Time to Bed_____ ☐ Spontaneous

Time Awake_____ Mood_____

Develop a bedtime routine. Was the dream incubated or spontaneous? Write down your mood.

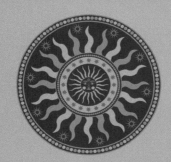

ARCHETYPES & IMAGES

On these pages you will list any images that stand out from your dream.

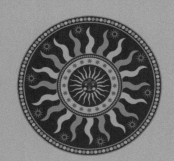

DREAM SKETCH

*Try making sketches of visual memories of the dream
in order to stimulate more details to memory.*

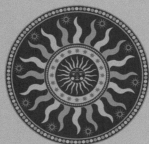

Return to this page after step four.

THE MEANING

*For this step include any understanding you have gained
as a result of examing your associations.*

_____
_____
_____
_____
_____
_____
_____
_____
_____
_____
_____
_____
_____
_____
_____
_____
_____
_____
_____
_____
_____
_____
_____
_____
_____
_____
_____
_____
_____
_____
_____
_____
_____
_____
_____
_____
_____
_____
_____
_____
_____

STEP THREE

Learning the Language of Your Dreams

I believe that every image in your dream has a special significance that belongs to you alone. In my own life, I have learned to greet my dream images, welcome them, and nurture them as my guests, and they have, in turn, elucidated and enriched my world. Based on this understanding, I have adapted an associative dreamwork method used by Jungian analyst Robert Johnson. Johnson believes that even when an image has an archetypal or universal meaning, it still has a personal connotation that one can only understand from within. An individual can uncover the significance of these images by examining the unconscious associations that arise in response to these images.

Our dreams show us parts of ourselves, some of which resist integration and others that desire to be seen. Sometimes these images can be disturbing or frightening to the conscious mind, but it is important to remember that they are symbolic and seldom literal. The images help us channel the unconscious parts of ourselves into consciousness so that we may interpret and integrate them.

Once we bring dream imagery into the conscious mind, the messages the images contain are always useful and intended to benefit the dreamer. We must learn to treat our dream images as companions that accompany us in two worlds - inner and outer. Sadly, our culture teaches us that only the external world has any importance. Once we align in affinity with our dreams, we begin to sense the tremendous power and intelligence behind them. Dreams can connect us to layers of ourselves that we long to know. They carry important themes that can illuminate a deepened experience of life and its meaning.

Accessing Associations: Step-by-Step

• After recording your dream at the end of this section; in the column opposite the "Archetypes and Images" column titled "Associations", write out the associations you have with each dream image. Dream imagery can include people (including your "dream self"), objects, situations, colors, sounds, or words.

• To come up with associations, take the images out of the context of the dream and ask yourself, "What feeling do I have about this image? What words or ideas come to mind when I think of it?" Jot down anything you spontaneously connect with the image, including feelings, memories, and mental pictures. For example, if you saw a frog in your dream, you might associate it with being bouncy, with a prince, with the color green, or with a particular time in your childhood. Meanwhile, if I dreamed of a frog, I might think of revulsion, fear, the jungle, or a tasty treat that was on the menu last night.

• Nothing is inconsequential at this phase. You are just gathering all of the intelligence you can from your own subconscious.

• As you explore your associations, don't go back to the dream for now. Just stick with the image by itself. You will notice that you will resonate with certain associations more deeply than others. Some associations may generate energy or activate parts of you that feel wounded or confused. Keep going, and don't try to make literal or rational sense of anything at this point.

• If you are not sure about an association, then move on to the following image. Allow as much space as you can for these associations. Keep your mind open, and don't force anything. Also, don't lock yourself into a singular meaning. Dreams and dream imagery can have multiple meanings that can all be true at once in our lives. Follow your intuition, and your understanding will grow as you move through the lessons and begin tying it all together.

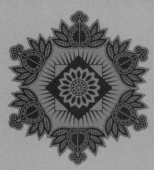

THE DREAM

Title_____

Write down your dream immediately upon waking and give it a title.

_____
_____
_____
_____
_____
_____
_____
_____
_____
_____
_____
_____
_____
_____
_____
_____
_____
_____
_____
_____
_____
_____
_____
_____
_____
_____
_____
_____
_____
_____
_____
_____
_____
_____
_____
_____
_____
_____
_____
_____
_____

Date_____ ☐ Incubated

Day of Week_____ or

Time to Bed_____ ☐ Spontaneous

Time Awake_____ Mood_____

Develop a bedtime routine. Was the dream incubated or spontaneous? Write down your mood.

ARCHETYPES & IMAGES

On this page you will list any images that stand out from your dream.

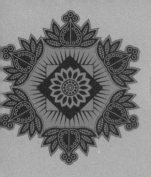

ASSOCIATIONS

On this page you will write out your associations to the corresponding images.

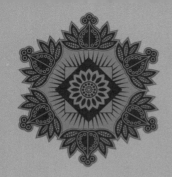

DREAM SKETCH

*Try making sketches of visual memories of the dream
in order to stimulate more details to memory.*

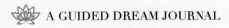

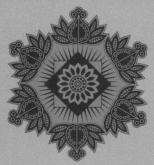

Return to this page after step four.

THE MEANING

For this step include any understanding you have gained as a result of examing your associations.

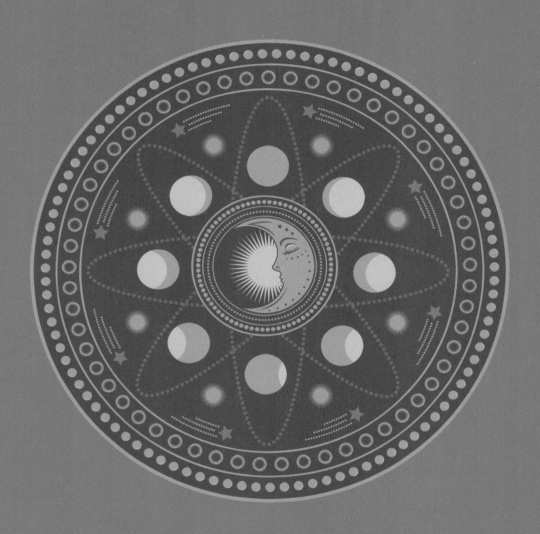

DREAMWORK for GROWTH & HEALING

STEP FOUR

Interpretation: Getting Answers

For this lesson, we will go back to our lists of images and associations from the previous section and begin working with them to open lines of communication and start getting answers. In my experience, dreams want us to wake up and pay attention. Through understanding and interpreting your own dream imagery, you have the opportunity to develop an intimate relationship with your dreams and connect to a powerful source of healing within yourself. Frequently, the information will be that which is not readily accessible to you in the waking world.

Dreams reflect the world and our relationship to our world. Dreams work to move us further along in our growth and evolution, and they capitalize on our natural creative capacity to deal with life's challenges. To interpret our dreams, we need to begin connecting the images in our dreams to the physical, emotional, and spiritual experiences in our waking lives. Most dreams reflect what is going on inside us: moral conflicts, stagnant energy, and unconscious patterns or memories that we are ready to integrate into our waking lives to our benefit.

Let's begin by dealing with the dream images you have collected, one by one. For each image, go through the associations you recorded and underline the ones that resonate most. For each image, ask yourself, "What part of me could this association refer to?" "What traits might I have in common with this image?" "What traits might I be missing?" "How are these characteristics showing up in my life?" "Are there traits in this image that I see in my own personality – either in the present or in the past?" Ask yourself, has this image shown up in an emotional way? Perhaps as an attitude or a mood? Where might I be feeling this way in my life? Remember to write everything down as you go.

If your image is an animal, in addition to any associations you have with the animal, consider that animals often represent primitive physical and instinctual energies. These instincts might point to a biological need for food or exercise or a desire for a sexual or sensual experience. During this phase, you might begin to feel strong resistance, particularly when dealing with distasteful images or characteristics. Allow these associations and dynamics to gently seep into your consciousness. Sometimes it may seem as though nothing is clicking; then, in a quiet moment, the understanding will come. Give yourself time, be patient, and allow space for contemplation.

Try thinking of each image/association as an individual character that exists inside you, a part of a greater whole. Get to know each image and its unique personality. Considering the characters this way will come in handy later when it is time to ritualize your understanding in the waking world. When you're working with an image and the association brings up intense emotions, you will feel a shift in your energy or sense some kind of reaction in your physical body; this is how you'll know you've made a connection. Intuition is a powerful tool as you do this work.

Here's an example:

Dream image: a cat

Associations - slinky, childhood pet, black, independent

The association that really clicks here is "independent." Ask yourself, "Where is that independent quality in me? Where am I independent? Where have I been independent in the past? Where do I want to be more independent in my life?" Perhaps you've been making decisions at work lately that you might categorize as independent. Or maybe you've been overly independent in an intimate relationship, and the image reflects this emotional distance. Questioning yourself in this way, you can begin to see how this image relates to an actual part of you and ascertain whether that image represents something in the present moment or a pattern from the past.

Interpretation

Next, find specific examples from your life that correspond with the qualities of each image. For instance, if your brother was in your dream and the characteristic you associated with your brother was his vanity or pride, you would want to look for where vanity or pride currently shows up in your life. Most of your dreams portray what is going on inside you rather than what is going on around you. The interpretation generally pertains to your personal journey toward wholeness. The collective unconscious simply borrows images and symbols from the external world to refer you back to something that needs to be revealed and seen in your inner world.

Because many images from the outside world may trigger this inner reflection, it can be tempting to take these images literally. This is particularly true when you are in conflict, in love, or in an emotional state of connection with the person who appears in your dream. However, we are better served by looking for the qualities in ourselves that our dreams offer us through images, rather than taking a literal approach and connecting these images to people or situations in our external world.

I'll use an example to demonstrate this literal vs. imaginal understanding. Let's say that I have a dream about my husband cheating on me with another woman. I could interpret this literally and wonder if this dream image is bringing up a trust issue or some doubt about our commitment or his loyalty. However, that's rarely, if ever, the case with a dream image like this. When I work through my associations with the image of my husband, I ask myself what qualities come to mind: innovative, provider, and father. I do the same for the woman in the dream, and I see that she represents sexiness, confidence, and a carefree spirit. When I connect these associations to parts of myself, I can see that the message in this dream image is really about recognizing my internal need to integrate my inner masculine and feminine characteristics. I might realize that I have lost track of some of my feelings about myself as a sexual being and have a desire to repossess them.

At this point, we can start to look at our dreams as mirrors in which all of our traits and characteristics appear if we're willing to look. We might see aspects of our personality about which we were not fully aware. We might discover that while it may be easy to negatively judge those who are carefree in their sexuality, this characteristic is actually something we also can possess and enjoy but have previously disallowed for various reasons.

We may not be ready to admit it now, but all of the traits that show up in our dreams exist somewhere inside us. This is not to say that dreams portray the traits literally, because dreams often use dramatic imagery or extremes to catch our attention. However, unlike the ego, the dream realm does not categorize things as "good" or "bad." It is worth considering that some traits that we might relegate to our Shadow or deem "negative" might be valuable to us when we bring them to a conscious level. Likewise, there is value in recognizing and living out the excellent qualities we find in ourselves.

Once you have a coherent statement of what the dream means as a whole, based on your associations, you can embark on the final task of interpretation. Your interpretation is complete when you tie your understanding of each of the images in the dream into a unified story that pertains to your life. As you can see with the above example, you might discover a central message, theme, or bit of advice once the story is complete. Whatever it is, it should flow out of the steps you have already followed: identifying the images, making the associations, and discovering the inner dynamics at play. The interpretation will not always be apparent immediately, but clarity can come more swiftly if you're already connected to your symbolic world. Think of the interpretation process as a puzzle.

As you continue to write out your ideas about the different puzzle pieces – dream images, associations, symbolic meanings – eventually, a clear, cohesive picture will come into view, and it will begin to make sense. Be willing to live with ambiguity for a while and be curious. To be sure that you are on the right track, ask yourself, "Is there something new here?" Assume that your dream has come to help you grow, wake up, change, or challenge old assumptions. It is also helpful to remember that the dreamworld auto-corrects. This means that if you should make an interpretation that is not 100% correct or miss something, there is no need to worry. The dream realm will present you with the information you need, as many times as it takes, to integrate it. Repetitive dreams serve to offer information over and over again. Both nightmares and repetitive dreams stop once you integrate the information held within them.

In the next few steps, we will explore how you can begin to incorporate and embody all the information your dreams share with you and use this information for your growth, health, happiness, and path to wholeness.

Practice: Go back to the previous three steps and make associations with the dream imagery you recorded. Next, underline the associations that you feel when holding the image in your mind (separate from the dream). Generally, we have an intuitive sense that we can also know in our body when we have hit on a meaningful association. Record a new dream following all of the steps through making meaning of the associations and your dream. You can use the "Meaning" pages provided.

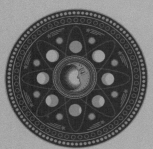

THE DREAM

Title_____

Write down your dream immediately upon waking and give it a title.

Date_____ ☐ Incubated

Day of Week_____ or

Time to Bed_____ ☐ Spontaneous

Time Awake_____· Mood_____

Develop a bedtime routine. Was the dream incubated or spontaneous? Write down your mood.

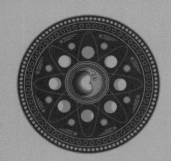

ARCHETYPES & IMAGES

On this page you will list any images that stand out from your dream.

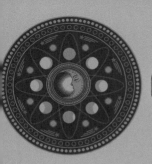

ASSOCIATIONS

On this page you will write out your associations to the corresponding images.

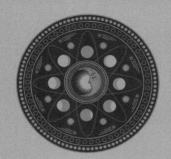

DREAM SKETCH

*Try making sketches of visual memories of the dream
in order to stimulate more details to memory.*

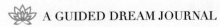

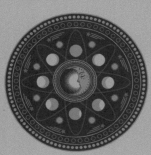

THE MEANING

*For this step include any understanding you have gained
as a result of examing your associations*

DREAMWORK for GROWTH & HEALING

STEP FIVE

Embodied Imagination®

In this lesson, I will introduce you to my all-time favorite dreamwork method. While I have already shared several helpful methods for working with your dreams, in this lesson, I will guide you to become embodied by the images themselves. Through Embodied Imagination, I will guide you to connect with the dream images through your body and connect with your sensory experience so that the images can share whatever insights or intelligence they have with you directly. Therefore, you will not need to interpret what the images represent because you will experience the unconscious wisdom connected to the images directly through your body's wisdom. You will feel it, know it, and anchor the wisdom in your body. You can use this method alone or in conjunction with the other techniques you have practiced.

Embodied Imagination (EI) is a therapeutic and creative method to work with dreams and memories pioneered by my teacher and mentor, Robert Bosnak. The method is based on principles first developed by Carl Jung, particularly on Jung's work on alchemy. EI is also based on the work of archetypal psychologist James Hillman. Embodied Imagination works with both dreams and memories and can be practiced individually or in groups, in psychotherapy, or with a certified EI practitioner. It is also used in medicine, theatre, art, and creative research. As a certified practitioner, I have adapted the practice for this journal.

During the practice of Embodied Imagination we return to the dreamworld's reality and explore its wisdom through direct experience. Embodied Imagination is a careful exploration of the creative imagination and unconscious realms. One achieves the embodied state through becoming fully immersed in the images that the dream environment presents. The dreamer shifts away from the ego's habitual perspective and gains access to the feelings, sensations, and intelligence of a variety of dream imagery perspectives. Working with imagery from this perspective stimulates an expanded state of consciousness that you can experience in your body. Embodied Imagination allows us to engage with and immerse ourselves in images that both nourish us and restore a sense of soul.

We will start to learn the Embodied Imagination practice beginning by using a memory. We all have access to memories, so we'll begin with a memory practice rather than using a dream. According to Dr. J.F. Pagel, a dream and consciousness scientist, memories (especially poignant ones) can be every bit as powerful as dreams. In my work with cancer patients, we often begin with memories instead of dreams. I found that exposure to the feelings associated with memory images helped them acknowledge feelings and fears that might not otherwise be manageable. Once the patients could see and feel some of the more challenging aspects of their diagnoses and treatment, they could recognize places that needed attention and take care of themselves in ways they hadn't considered before. In my experience, the most compelling information and insights in dreamwork often come from the images that we find the most disagreeable or alien. This is a rich place of discovery. Be daring.

Embodied Imagination Practice: Let's start by searching for a potent memory image. The memory can be from any time or experience, positive or negative; just make sure to pick one that has a good strong feeling tone. Again, I encourage feeling your way into this as we want a memory and associated image that has life to it (a memory that includes smells, sounds, emotions, etc.). Which memories are attractive or interesting to you? Which ones repel you? Now would be a good time to recall that the memory image we are looking for is not literal (think of it as an archetype). Sometimes, the images that repel the day-to-day you (your habitual consciousness) may carry a completely different charge in the subconscious. The idea is to "re-enter" the memory in a dream-like state.

STEP FIVE

Once you have chosen your image, revisit the memory in your mind, placing yourself inside the memory as if it were happening right now. Next, think about your associations with this memory image. Take your time with this as it is an important step to re-familiarize yourself with the memory and place it in context.

Next, we will prepare to re-enter and relive the memory to connect with the wisdom and perspective inside the image. This is a very precise process. We must approach it slowly, carefully, respectfully, and without expectations. Whenever you hear your rational mind narrating or hijacking the process (often with the words "I think"), go back to the image and notice precisely what is there physically.

Part of the preparation to re-enter the memory is doing a body scan. Beginning with a body scan will allow you to relax and will bring you into a hypnogogic state – the state between waking and sleeping – which is ideal for dream recall. This state will also allow you to have a baseline for noticing any changes that come about once you have become embodied by an image. Once you are embodied, you will constantly be aware both of the experience of the image and the fact that you are safely and comfortably in a room practicing Embodied Imagination. Embodied Imagination is a state of dual consciousness. There is no map or guidebook for this excursion, and we never know in advance what these images will hold. This is an exercise in trusting your not-knowing enough to allow the intelligence of something new to emerge. We all have access to memories. So we'll begin with a memory practice rather than using a dream.

On the following page you will find a step-by-step guide for a body scan. Once you've completed the body scan, you will begin recreating your memory as an imagined environment; then, you will become embodied by the memory image; finally, you will share a perspective with the image and anchor the experience in your body so that you can reference it later. The entire process should take around 20-30 minutes if you include writing time. This will be the same process that you will use for embodying dream images.

Practice: Body Scan

Start by finding a comfortable position, either sitting or lying down, close your eyes, and focus inward. Next, bring your attention to a spot at the center of the top of your head and feel your own warm intention to relax as you descend through your body, simply noticing how it is in this current moment, without changing a thing; envision a ball filled with this intention. Then, simply allow this ball to drop down into your head. Notice the state of your head, inside and out, notice the temperature... moisture... tension... softness... movement... just notice without any intention to change anything. Imagine you are giving your head a warm bath with your attention. Descend through the neck and shoulders... arms and hand... into the chest and back... all following the same slow and attentive process. Continue this process descending all the way to the soles of the feet. Include every part of you in between. As you come to the soles of your feet, you likely now feel quite relaxed and ready to begin exploring your image.

Transitioning to Embodiment:

• When working with an image, slow down. Avoid rushing. Get extremely precise. You will find deeper sensations and emotions embedded in the image by slowing down and noticing the details.

• As you approach an image, notice the environment. Where are you? What is around you? What do you see, smell, feel, hear? How far are you from the image? What is the lighting like? What is the temperature? Etc.

• If you choose to explore and embody a "dream you," begin by noticing things like your age, your clothing, and your posture. Be sure to stick with what the image is showing you, rather than what your habitual or ego-consciousness thinks about what you're seeing.

• Focusing on the eyes (or other intense qualities) of an image can often be a good place to sense into that image's perspective and make the transition into feeling it yourself. Allow yourself to be absorbed. Eventually, after noticing the finer details of the image, you may begin to try sensing into what it is like to be the image, sense into what it is feeling. Sometimes, physically mimicking a posture or adjusting your breathing can be helpful at this stage. What does it feel like to be in a body that moves this way?

Anchoring the image:

• Anchoring helps the dreamer imprint the emotional, felt experience of the image in the body. Once an experience is anchored in your body, then it can be integrated into your waking consciousness.

• Finding the anchor requires participation in the image's state, both physical and emotional. Once you are aware of the image's perspective and emotional state, pinpoint exactly where you feel it in your body and what the sensation is like.

• Once you connect to the sensation in your body that's associated with the image, continue to anchor it there for a minute or so. For example, if you become aware that an image feels quite spacious and peaceful, then note where you feel this peaceful sensation in your body. Let's say you feel this sense of space and peace in the heart. Take a few moments and really sense into that peace and spaciousness in your heart, allowing it to settle in the body. Once you have anchored the embodiment, you can later practice and access its particular qualities as needed.

When you practice embodiment, the image conveys a palpable experience uniquely suited to you. The insight, or catharsis, or joy, or healing that you may experience results from participating in a mutual state with entities that in some way belong to you and vice versa.

Using Embodied Imagination as a tool for guidance in the dream realm is a powerful practice. You can also use Embodied Imagination to incubate your concerns into the dream environment to elicit a response. Find an image associated with your question or concern and then deeply inhabit and embody it (specifically: the feeling of it) for a few seconds before you drift off to sleep. Once you've done this, remember to set your intention or write it down in your dream journal. Review Lesson 2 if you need help with this practice.

The incubation process paves the way for visitation by a dream, which will infuse you with its intelligence through the process of Embodied Imagination. When we encounter images in a dream, we must approach them with the understanding that they are preparing our consciousness to move forward and to transform from the inside out. These images are excellent advisors and allow us a safe environment to examine a variety of perspectives. In our dreams, we encounter allies, and it is our task to simply ask for their assistance and honor what they show us.

"What I have found after more than a decade of researching, examining, exploring, and analyzing dreams – of others as well as my own – is that most circumstances in people's lives have a long unconscious history that can be perceived and integrated through the dream realm once the awareness is present to do so."

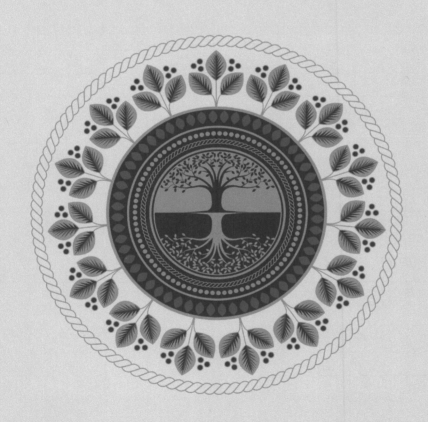

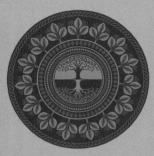

THE DREAM

Title_____

Write down your dream immediately upon waking and give it a title.

Date_____   ☐ Incubated

Day of Week_____   or

Time to Bed_____   ☐ Spontaneous

Time Awake_____   Mood_____

Develop a bedtime routine. Was the dream incubated or spontaneous? Write down your mood.

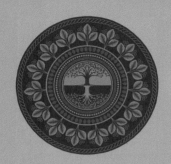

ARCHETYPES & IMAGES

On this page you will list any images that stand out from your dream.

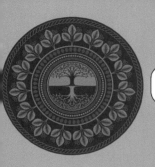

ASSOCIATIONS

On this page you will write out your associations to the corresponding images.

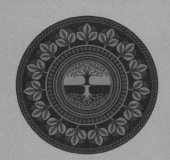

DREAM SKETCH

*Try making sketches of visual memories of the dream
in order to stimulate more details to memory.*

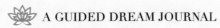

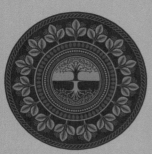

THE MEANING

*For this step include any understanding you gained
as a result of embodiment.*

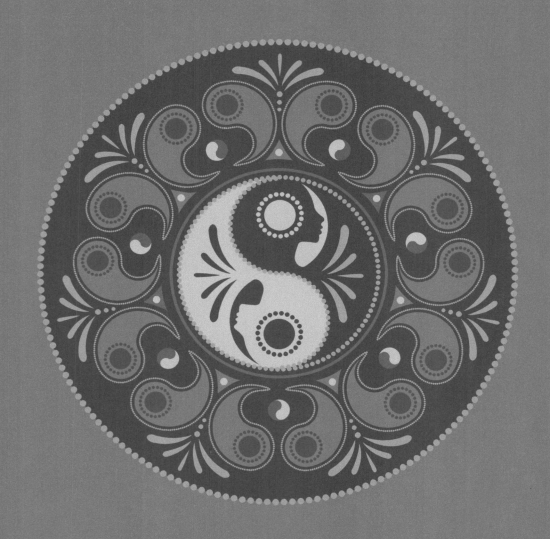

DREAMWORK for GROWTH & HEALING

STEP SIX

Integration and Healing

A foundational order in the psyche unifies the assorted archetypes. According to Jung, this central archetype of wholeness is the Self. The Self is defined through a conscious and healthy relationship with the divine symbols and imagery of the unconscious. As I have come into relationship with my dreams, these unconscious symbols have been my guides. Through focus and determination, and hours of stillness and listening, they've come to guide me in my waking life as well. These symbols are teachers and parents that I never had, lovers and protectors; they are my wounded inner child and the heroine that I have become. I hope, in time, the same will be true for you.

The process of finding meaning in my wounds and challenges through dreamwork, as well as through counseling others, has been incredibly healing and inspirational. I have come to embrace the idea that if you listen to and work with the unconscious, the psyche, in turn, will work with and for you. As archetypal psychologist James Hillman so beautifully stated, "Attention is the cardinal psychological virtue. On it depends perhaps the other cardinal virtues, for there can hardly be faith nor hope nor love for anything unless it first receives attention." As you come into relationship with your dreams and imagery, you will have many new insights, new dreams, and a changed understanding of yourself, your personality structure, and the way forward. Now, rather than saying, "I had a dream," you may begin to feel that you and the dream are becoming one.

In my experience, even the worst dreams can bring meaning to our existence. The events and challenges you deal with in your day-to-day life often have deep roots in the unconscious. Once you establish a willingness and aptitude to attend to what the unconscious shows you through your dreams, these roots can be seen, honored, and integrated. I believe that dream images, which can be considered archetypal due to the value you give them, can help you accept yourself with more kindness and understanding and can open pathways for you to evolve, grow, and heal. They will allow you to love and trust in ways that may have seemed unfathomable before.

Dreams are a threshold into the unconscious from the conscious, ego state. As we slog through the muck toward balance and wholeness, we must accept confrontation along the way. Finding wholeness means reconciling opposites – the fundamental opposites being the split between the conscious and unconscious. The experience of knowing the Self creates wholeness. Sometimes the waking ego prefers less complicated views of itself and reality, and it takes some time and some nudging to be moved from its perspective. Ego is the 'I' we think of when we think of our identity in the first person. Dreams maintain an objectivity that provides that which is necessary for psychic balance, regardless of the ego's wishes. Dream images and symbolic experiences in your outer life are the means by which the unconscious confronts the ego. The chaotic sensations that go along with such encounters are necessary for growth. The conscious and the unconscious must frequently enter into a confrontation to find balance.

Fortunately, dreams can provide us with access to helpful dynamics that we may lack in our ego-based waking state. The ego is merely the tip of the iceberg that can be seen above the surface. The more substantial part of the iceberg that remains hidden underneath, and the depth of the ocean surrounding it, is the unconscious mind.

Poet-philosopher Rainer Maria Rilke explained this dynamic beautifully to a young man who was anxious and insecure: "We have no reason to distrust our world, for it is not against us. Has it terrors, they are our terrors; has it abysses, those abysses belong to us; are dangers at hand, we must try to love them. And if only we arrange our life according to that principle which counsels us that we must always hold to the difficult, then that which now still seems to us the most alien will become what we most trust and find most faithful."

Dream interpretation facilitates growth and healing by supplementing the dreamer's conscious experiences with patterns and symbols from the unconscious realm. There is a delineation between what is above the water's surface and what is hidden below; this split is the barrier to wholeness. When the unconscious realm seeps into our awareness through the images and symbols in our dreams, repressed energies are released, and there is an opening for the unconscious to come through and mend the psychic split between the two worlds. For the hidden potential in these images and symbols to be revealed, the messages must be acknowledged, honored, and valued by the conscious mind. Then, your next step toward integration and wholeness becomes clear.

There is a reason that we spend one-third of our lives asleep. We sleep and dream to reconnect with the soulful aspects of our psyche that arise from the depths of our unconscious and be reenergized by them. This reconnective healing process restores and balances our conscious mind. The primary purpose for remembering dreams is to gain access to facets of our psyche so that we can benefit from assimilating and integrating them into our waking consciousness. Our dream lives are not controlled by the conscious mind, so they reveal an inner truth that reflects reality as it is, not as we would like it to be. It is as though the psyche does not wish to continue the tensions of waking life but wants to resolve them, recover from them, and thrive as a result.

While some of our dreams' contents may pass from our minds or be repressed from conscious experiences into the unconscious, Jung hypothesized that all psychic contents, including dreams, have their roots in the collective unconscious. This hypothesis assumes that all behaviors and perceptions must be within an individual's potential realm before they can become actual. All of these potentialities are contents within the collective unconscious.

With the help of dreams, you can begin to recognize certain archetypes from the collective. For example, elements of Shadow are repressed qualities, not admitted or accepted because they are incompatible with what we believe about ourselves. By recognizing this, we begin to make the Shadow conscious. Expressing the Shadow consciously and accepting its qualities requires great care and can be disturbing. Still, it holds the potential for breaking outdated ways of seeing ourselves and our traits. Often, the images we find most disgusting or perverse in dreams are precisely the ones that can restore us to the powerful, pristine, and numinous person we were always meant to be.

Example: Let's examine a dream in which you see your husband with a lover. Upon looking more deeply, we might discover that the mind associates the woman in the dream with judgmental ideas about promiscuity and/or sexual freedom. Upon deeper reflection, however, we might discover that this quality is, in fact, one that you desire more in your own life. The woman, in this case, is a representation of Shadow, and honest and open analysis can allow for conscious integration. Get ready for your new wild and free sex life!

The Divine or Wounded Child archetype can be found in dreams, inner experiences, and day-to-day life and is an image that individuals carry throughout their lives. The Wounded Child is the part of the human personality that wants to develop and become whole. Therefore, take note when children show up in your dreams. Recently, an older woman client without children came in with a dream she found quite strange because, in it, she held and was cuddling a newborn baby. She felt quite protective of this baby, and felt like there were others in the dream who wanted to harm it. When we reviewed this dream in light of her associations with both the "dream her" and the baby, it became clear that the dream was a response to the psychotherapeutic work we had been doing. She was in the process of loving and nurturing back into the world, a part of herself that had been neglected as a child. She was reassured by this dream that she could and would reclaim those parts of her that were associated with the baby. According to Jung, each of us has this eternal child within us, part of us that is constantly becoming – it calls for unceasing care, attention, and education.

I consider coming into relationship with your dreams to be a kind of journey. Like a heroine's journey, dreamwork begins as an inner calling that manifests when experiences appear to indicate that one must face or do something. This calling can feel like a deep longing for something, even if that 'something' remains unknown. Eventually, a response arises in a dream, and the dreamer must find the courage to face the unknown. As we move between worlds and states of being – between the known and the unknown, the conscious and the unconscious – the images and symbols guide us along our way. We return from this journey knowing more about ourselves and having a deeper sense of the immense worlds that exist within us.

Hosting my dream images has allowed me to reanimate my life. In my unconscious realm, I have seen a mute and terrorized Child, a profoundly critical Devouring Mother, a murderous Demon Trickster, and an erotic, confused Femme Fatale archetype, among many others. I learned to personify them and to love them. In this way, I faced what was hidden in my heart and soul and allowed myself to see it as part of my Self.

As you proceed with this important work, I wish you courage, curiosity, and fortitude. Remember that all of this work is in service of bringing to light your best and most integrated Self.

As you work through these steps to understand and integrate dreams for growth and healing, remember: each dream involves an implicit question. The question might be regarding the meaning behind your symptoms of depression or anxiety, or it might be a question that helps you discover which archetype is expressing itself in your current reality (that you might emulate for your brightest future). By addressing these questions, we become active instead of passive participants in life's ups and downs. Our inner worlds cluster around charged energies, complexes, and past experiences that haven't been fully understood or integrated. Virtually anything in the outer world can activate these unconscious energy patterns that are constantly swirling beneath the surface - waiting to be revealed and then healed.

This is particularly true in our intimate relationships. When these charged energies emerge as a result of some external force, we must make a conscious effort to change our perspective, or these patterns will control us, and we will continue to react in unconscious ways. Through dreamwork, you will gain an enhanced capacity for empathy and a new perspective based on the remembrance of earlier times - times in life when vulnerability was possible, and love was welcome. Our most intimate relationships - with lovers, children, family, or even therapists - are the most accurate mirrors for our lives and offer us the greatest opportunity for healing.

For all of us, loving and freeing the Divine Child lost within can be a part of the quest that gives life meaning. Incredible growth comes from uniting the unconscious aspects of that vulnerable child with a protector that we've never had. By bringing these aspects to light, the Child can learn to trust, love, and live again as a whole Self. It is essential to recognize that the vulnerable child, and the protector whom the child comes to trust, are both within you. There is no external protector who can provide this for you – you are both the vulnerable child and the loving parent. You are supported in this journey, and you can always seek external support if you need it, but the journey to wholeness takes place within you. By consciously acknowledging the need for a protector, you can embark on the path to wholeness with a thirst for meaning as your companion. From this perspective, I view both the road in front of you and that behind you as a Hero/Heroine's journey.

Joseph Campbell, the American mythologist and writer, recounted that having traversed the threshold, the hero moves in a dream landscape of "curiously fluid, ambiguous forms, where he must survive a succession of trials." Here, the hero discovers for the first time that a benign power is everywhere, supporting him in his passage. I discovered the presence of a benign power supporting me through my own healing and in all aspects of my life through my analyst's guidance and through thoroughly exploring my dreams. I learned that I could risk reimagining infinite possibilities in the world, as a child might, and that the psyche provides whatever is necessary along our path if only we take the time to lovingly attend to the numinous images within. I hope that you will embrace this journey and enjoy numerous discoveries along the way for yourself.

This is not necessarily a journey that one must take alone. I could have never done some parts of it alone. If you encounter difficulty integrating or managing anything that comes up due to this work, I encourage you to seek someone out to support you – a therapist, coach, family member, friend, or dream group.

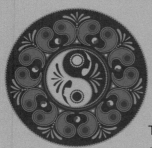

THE DREAM

Title_____

Write down your dream immediately upon waking and give it a title.

_____
_____
_____
_____
_____
_____
_____
_____
_____
_____
_____
_____
_____
_____
_____
_____
_____
_____
_____
_____
_____
_____
_____
_____
_____
_____
_____
_____
_____
_____
_____
_____
_____
_____
_____
_____

Date_____   ☐ Incubated

Day of Week_____   or

Time to Bed_____   ☐ Spontaneous

Time Awake_____   Mood_____

Develop a bedtime routine. Was the dream incubated or spontaneous? Write down your mood.

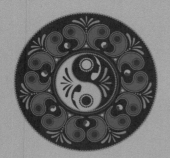

ARCHETYPES & IMAGES

On this page you will list any images that stand out from your dream.

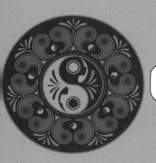

ASSOCIATIONS

On this page you will write out your associations to the corresponding images.

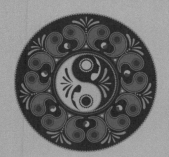

DREAM SKETCH

*Try making sketches of visual memories of the dream
in order to stimulate more details to memory.*

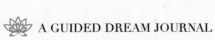

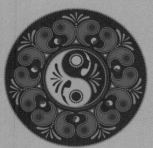

THE MEANING

*For this step include any understanding you gained
as a result of analyzing your dream.*

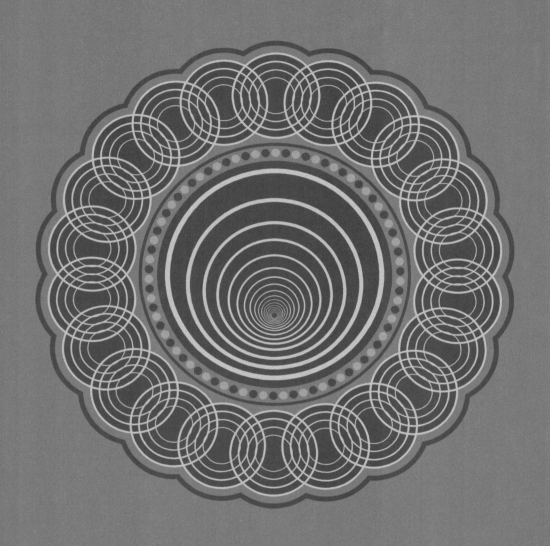

DREAMWORK for GROWTH & HEALING

STEP SEVEN

Keeping the Dream Alive

According to physicist and philosopher Luc Sala, ritual exists in every part of our daily lives. We find rituals at work, in religion, in relationships, and in schools. We use rituals to ease the mind, help us concentrate, aid with meditation and focus, and express gratitude. We can also use ritual to connect deeply with ourselves, which is how we can more easily access metaphysical dimensions such as the dream realm. Ritual is a bridge to connect us to the magic and the fire that we all possess within. For these reasons and more, Sala refers to ritual as "practical magic."

In Western culture, ritual is not as woven into the thread of daily life and doesn't have the same meaning that it does in other cultures. While rituals are commonly found in medicine and psychiatry, such as professionals wearing white lab coats or particular seating arrangements (which undoubtedly create a placebo effect for patients, based on beliefs and expectations), these rituals do not get credit for helping us deal with life's pitfalls and crises. Some religious rituals originally intended, designed, and understood to be magically effective, have lost their deeper purpose and have become more ceremonial, having lost the fabric of meaning instilled with faith as the foundation.

Ritual differs from ceremony; ceremony is bound to social and psychological constructs, while ritual intends to influence and interact with the metaphysical realm. Ritual offers us a means of affecting both internal and external reality by joining the two. Ritual uses particular processes and magical links as a special means for correspondence. This correspondence then reflects into our ordinary waking reality, much like a bridge between the waking self we associate with "reality" and a (perhaps more comprehensive) reality known as the dream realm. Often the results of this correspondence and the messages we receive are not rational or logical.

Ritual has evolved over time, and the magical aspects have been lost or replaced by more "objective" practices. Recently, however, many people show a growing interest in shamanism, ancestral wisdom, and the rituals of various tribal cultures. We have lost our sense of ritual's psychological and spiritual role in our lives, but our instinctual hunger for meaningful ritual remains. We have begun to rediscover ritual as a natural human tool for connecting to our inner selves. Letting go of the ego, stepping out of the small self, and getting in touch with a deeper self are all core to the process of reconnecting to ritual in our everyday lives.

Developing Rituals to Honor Our Dreams

The next step in our dreamwork requires a physical act that will concretize and integrate the dream's message into our waking lives. This act or ritual might be a practical act, such as following instructions that you have received from the dream realm in your waking life, or it could be a symbolic act such as offering a gift to the archetypal Child in your dream to facilitate deeper communication and understanding.

Once you've interpreted the dream, then it's time to actively work with the interpretation. It helps to use your imagination when crafting these rituals since imagination and dreams come from the same source. Give your imagination and the dream time together in your mind. This final step can significantly enhance your understanding of the dream and help to bring any necessary changes into form.

Don't get stuck trying to come up with extensive or elaborate rituals. Any ritual will serve you as long as it corresponds with the dream's message. We want the dream to register deeply with the unconscious. Therefore you might carry out your ritual silently and alone, like a prayer, or in some other, more public manner, such as beginning to sing aloud in front of others or displaying a painting you've created. Ritual in dreamwork brings your dream down to Earth and into the reality of your day-to-day life. We use big and small symbolic acts to bridge the unconscious mind and the conscious world. This bridge goes two ways, and a consciously conducted ritual will send a potent message back to the dream realm communicating our willingness to change. When we send this message of our willingness back to the places where our attitudes and behaviors originated, we can create profound change and open a doorway to growth and healing.

This communication unlocks stagnant energy that can eventually be available to us so that we may create on a conscious level. It is necessary to get both our minds and our bodies involved so that the intelligence in our dreams moves from a theoretical level to a gut-level understanding. Similar to the Embodied Imagination practice from Step Four, you need to initiate a physical action in your day-to-day life for the dream to become fully integrated with your waking reality.

In my own journey with dreamwork, I have developed many rituals. Over time, I came to recognize the Wounded Child archetype within me. Some of the ways I would interact with her in my waking reality would be to go out and buy her a doll or write a poem about how she looked as I held her in the dream. My dreams showed me that my Wounded Child needed to be nurtured and have her feelings of abandonment acknowledged, which was part of my wholeness journey. The actions I took with her in my waking life were inspired by the messages she showed me in the dream realm. Sometimes, in enacting these rituals, grief would arise, which was a healing act of compassion and empathy in itself.

I am careful not to suggest rituals when working with clients, as I feel they must come from the dreamer. We will often review what a client believes the dream is sharing based on our work. Sometimes it will be apparent to them what the dream is sharing as a whole, or (particularly when using the Embodied Imagination practice) they will have strong feelings about the intelligence held within individual images within the dream. In either case, the next question is always, "So, how are you going to make that real in the here and now?" The idea is to impress upon the conscious mind what you learned from the unconscious. You want to stay with the dream, work with the messages in your waking life, and take things one step at a time – this work is about what is happening INSIDE you. We want to allow our dreams a chance to manifest both inwardly and outwardly so that we may become aware of subtle connections that help us to see where the two worlds meet.

Exercise:

For this step, I would like you to conduct a ritual honoring your understanding of a recent dream. Take note of how performing the ritual makes you feel. Here are some considerations for coming up with your dream rituals:

• Keep your physical rituals small and subtle, and they will be more powerful. Discover the inner shift in perspective or attitude that presents itself through the dream imagery – acceptance, clarity, compassion – and then make the ritual a physical representation of that change.

• Contemplate how you can impress the principles learned from the unconscious realm upon the conscious mind.

• Ask yourself: "What is the essence of the fundamental truth the dream is trying to teach me? What is the essence of the archetypal energy in the dream?"

• Tap into your imagination to discover the ritual that will best serve to honor a particular dream or image. Accept whatever comes. Try not to conduct your ritual around the literal figures in your dream. Focus your ritual on the parts of YOURSELF symbolized by the dream images or your understanding of what the dream shared based on your analysis from

Step Three.

  • If you can't come up with something that relates directly to your dream, just come up with a physical act in honor of the dream, such as lighting a candle, lighting incense, or playing music while you consciously consider the dream. These acts will also register with the unconscious.

  • Allow your rituals to express your gratitude, elation, or awe. Sometimes, we can also use a ritual to express our fear, giving it a voice or a place in our consciousness that is both manageable and safe.

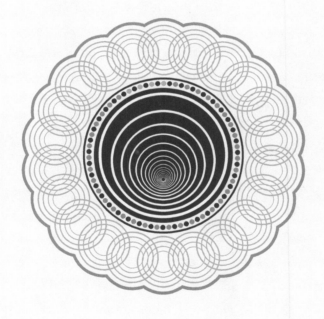

CONCLUSION

Right around the time I decided to pursue a Master's degree in Depth Psychotherapy, I began seeing a psychotherapist, both as a requirement of my program and to make sense of my life. Once we started working with my dreams, new dreams would come, each holding a new bit of information about where I was wounded. I began to grieve, to have empathy for myself, and to heal. In one cathartic dreamwork session, I finally faced the Daemon murderer in my dreams, after which he never returned. I came to understand him as a signpost. Wherever he showed up in dreams, there was something beyond the terror he caused me that I needed to recognize and integrate into my waking world. I believe he came into being when I was a child to turn me away from things that would have been simply too much to bear. He was the dream counterpart of dissociation.

Dissociation can sometimes protect the psyche against the damaging impact of trauma. Life can proceed because dissociation breaks up the intolerable experience and distributes it to different compartments of the mind and body, especially the 'unconscious' aspects of mind and body. Dreamwork can promote healing by mending the split between our waking lives and the unconscious. In the end, I am grateful that the Daemon murderer was able to be in service to my psyche in this way.

Over time, I learned about the different archetypes that arose in response to my suffering and will to survive. There was the Party Girl, the Femme Fatale, and Ariadne who came out in a fairytale I wrote, searching for Mother and saved by a Mermaid. Later came the Wounded Child, The Wounded Healer, The Warrior Princess, and the Spider Woman. Only recently, I have begun dreaming of capable, talented, and enchanting men, as well as myself as a hermaphrodite. These archetypes pave the way for my progress along my journey, but only once I acknowledge and tend to them with love and respect do they make the path less difficult. During difficult times, I find it helpful to remind myself of all of the archetypal defenses that I have integrated and that are still accessible to me. There is always more work to do.

Dreaming is an essential part of the human experience in virtually every culture on Earth There are references and documentation regarding dreams going back throughout recorded history within the world's vast array of religious and spiritual traditions, including mysticism and shamanism. Many of the earliest human communities included shamans, who not only served as healers but intervened between the living and the dead using dreams and visions.

The soul, as expressed in dreams by way of collective imagery, understands our needs and will generate dreams that elevate us beyond our suffering. The same is true for frustrations and unmet desires. Dreams compensate by showing us strength in the face of weakness, abundance in the face of poverty, and health when confronted by sickness. This natural and reciprocal process creates a balance that allows us to move in a desired direction. In other words, the dream shows us the opposite experience, emotion, or circumstance to give us perspective on the duality of the human experience. This natural process of dreaming sows hope in the face of temporary powerlessness and can catalyze action and movement when required.

Dreams arrange themselves so that we can uncover and begin to utilize our gifts and talents in daily life. Dreams fulfill a natural and universal function. Everyone dreams, and it is up to us to turn dreaming into an inspiring, supportive, and stimulating activity. Gratitude is also necessary to understand or heal whatever emotions or parts of ourselves we reveal. By thanking our dreams in advance for the gifts to come, we validate our capacity to receive. We are souls with unlimited potential, and dreams help us to realize this fully and express this power of creation in our waking world.

Finally, just as we encourage our dreams with our attention, we can also encourage them with others' attention. Dream sharing can become a rewarding social activity, leading to all kinds of new experiences and interactions. Dream sharing with a friend or family member is a great way to connect and practice your dream skills with someone else's dream images. Children LOVE sharing their dreams, but our culture rarely gives them a chance to do so. Once you've practiced using associations to glean meaning from your own dreams, why not give it a try with someone else's? Perhaps one day, we might return to an understanding that we make contact with our souls through dreamwork, and dream healing sanctuaries might spring up again around the world. Perhaps then, intellect and knowing can enter into dialogue with other ways of knowing to allow for a more collaborative lifestyle appropriate for the world in which we live.

Until then, Sweet Dreams.

"We must learn how to go into the unconscious realm known as dreaming and become receptive to its messages. This process of self-discovery can be accomplished through hosting and attending to our dreams and the personally meaningful images they hold."

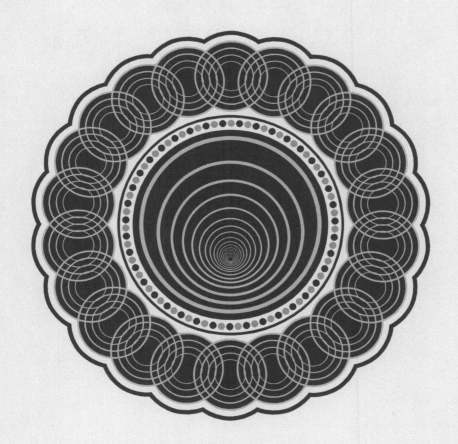

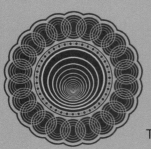

THE DREAM

Title_____

Write down your dream immediately upon waking and give it a title.

Date _____   ☐ Incubated

Day of Week _____   or

Time to Bed _____   ☐ Spontaneous

Time Awake _____   Mood _____

Develop a bedtime routine. Was the dream incubated or spontaneous? Write down your mood.

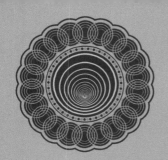

ARCHETYPES & IMAGES

*On this page you will list any images that stand
out from your dream.*

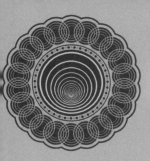

ASSOCIATIONS

On this page you will write out your associations to the corresponding images.

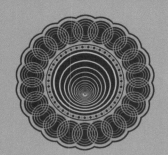

DREAM SKETCH

*Try making sketches of visual memories of the dream
in order to stimulate more details to memory.*

DREAMWORK for GROWTH & HEALING

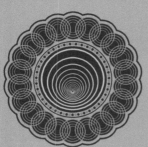

THE MEANING

For this step include any understanding you gained as a result of analyzing your dream.

GROUNDED IN SCIENCE

With modern technology, we can observe changes in the brain and apply neuroscience to the study of dreaming to provide a further understanding of how dreamwork and Embodied Imagination can be beneficial to our growth and healing. In his assessment of neurocognitive theories of dreaming, world-renowned dream researcher Richard Domhoff examined findings on dream development, including adult dream content and the neural substrates that subserve dreaming. He noted that the social networks in dreams are quite similar to those in waking life. They have properties also found in memory networks and in many aspects of the social and natural worlds. In other words, dreams are much more organized and intentional than was previously thought. The most recent research shows that brain activity patterns that represent images in our dreams are created by reactivating the patterns originally produced when we saw similar images in waking life.

Further research has shown that the main differences between waking and dreaming experiences relate to reality orientation and logical organization. This indicates that dreaming is not really impaired but simply monitors reality differently; dreamers experience their dreams as real. Research focused on the neural and cognitive processes that support imagining or simulating future events found that dreaming involves a subset of thought processes that imaginatively place the individual in a hypothetical scenario. This means we explore potential outcomes in our sleep! As Domhoff put it, "dreams can be characterized as 'embodied' simulations in the strict psychological sense of the term as off-line cognition that is body based." As many people seem to process the traumas they experience in their waking lives through the images in their dreams, recreating these dreaming experiences might build on dream embodiment in ways that benefit the dreamer.

Neuroscientists report that sleep disruptions that occur early after trauma exposure associate with an increased risk for post-traumatic stress disorder (PTSD), adding further insight to the understanding of sleep and dreaming. Domhoff described an emotional brain function that may be the basis for the PTSD nightmare. Researchers also point out that the strong emotional tone of mental activity during sleep garners speculation that we process difficult emotions in our dreams.

Recent research examining the re-emergence of sleep symptoms, including nightmares and disturbing dreams, coinciding with the COVID-19 pandemic, supports earlier findings that these sleep symptoms may be early warning signs of the sympathetic activation and arousal modulation seen in PTSD. Researchers note that attending to these dreams and nightmares could have useful implications for treatment and prevention for those who may be a high risk for developing PTSD, such as front-line workers. Considering the epidemic (at the time of this writing) of COVID-19, a life-threatening illness, future research might also examine the value of viewing these workers' dreams as possible precursors to PTSD and dreamwork as a potential tool to treat symptoms before or as they occur.

According to the continuity hypothesis of dreams, one's dreams reflect the events of one's waking days. Research results indicate a direct connection between dream imagery and health issues, including emotional health. Dreamwork connects dream imagery directly to the dreamer's waking life in relevant and meaningful ways. Given this continuity hypothesis, it would only seem natural that people's dreams would begin to reflect their concern regarding COVID-19 or any other impactful events in their lives.

The continuity hypothesis does not follow Jung's theory that dreams serve a compensatory function. However, when considering dreamwork and Jung's theories as I have applied them in this journal, I do not find that Jung's theories and the continuation hypothesis need to be mutually exclusive. During dreamwork, images that appear as a continuation of a traumatic life circumstance during waking experience frequently hold states or associations that benefit the dreamer; therefore, both continuation and compensation co-occur.

Research examining the continuity between waking mood and dream emotions found that the waking mood has an effect on dreams and that dreams featuring emotional intensity affect subsequent daytime waking mood! This lends support to the idea that working with a dream may impact the dreamer's waking experience. Frequently, images that might initially appear as negative, or that cause emotional distress, prove to be useful once the dreamer explores and embodies their associations. Dreamers can then access beneficial physical and emotional traits that were not consistently accessible before working with the dream.

Psychologists examining university students' dreams during the onset of COVID-19 found that these students' dream imagery had many more associations related to anxiety and the virus than that of a control group that provided dreams recorded before the pandemic. This finding is consistent with previous studies suggesting that waking-day anxiety carries over into dreaming. Due to the continued presence of COVID-19, many people (at the time of this writing) currently experience illness, job loss, isolation from family and friends, and grief and fear.

As all people face this life-threatening illness, and these concerns reflect not only in their waking hours but also in dreams, I suggest that practicing dreamwork with COVID-19 dreams might help alleviate the associated stress and anxiety. Individuals can learn and practice dreamwork at a distance using videoconferencing platforms such as Zoom. Therefore, trained dreamwork practitioners can readily conduct training in dreamwork methods, even during social distancing.

Dream researchers discovered a potentially functional connection between dreaming and emotional trauma recovery in divorced women who suffered depression; this functional connection may relate to current elevated anxiety. After one year, the women who had the most frequent and emotionally intense dreams featuring their ex-spouses were most likely to be in remission from depression. Further research showed a potentially causal interaction between sleep and emotional brain function. Researchers found that people with mood disorders also displayed sleep abnormalities in the brain during Rapid Eye Movement (REM) sleep. Additionally, they found that REM sleep decreased next-day reactivity to waking emotional experiences. This research highlights and supports the value of processing and integrating the emotional content held by dream imagery.

One of my teachers, psychologist and parapsychologist Dr. Stanley Krippner, describes nightmares as frightening and memorable dreams that frequently awaken the dreamer and are characterized by unpleasant emotions such as grief and terror. He notes that PTSD nightmares can persist throughout life, long after the other trauma symptoms resolve. He recommends that nightmare modification may be vital to resolve PTSD and aid the traumatized individual in recovery.

He claims that "as long as the PTSD nightmare recurs, the dreamer of the nightmare is blocked from resolving basic existential conflicts that prevent him or her from moving ahead." This recommendation for nightmare modification is in line with dreamwork's benefits, as I have witnessed them, as nightmares and repetitive dreams do not generally return once the individual integrates the information held in the dream. As Krippner notes, "PTSD is a consequence of modern life," and PTSD nightmares are devastating to those who experience them. These findings indicate the need for future research examining the benefits of revisiting nightmares using dreamwork practices.

Results from other studies suggest a core correlate of conscious emotional experiences during sleep. In further support of the proposed similarities in brain processing during dreams and waking life, neuropsychiatry researchers found that dreaming subjects' brain activity linked visual areas and areas used to integrate the senses. Additionally, a sleep study found that taking a nap blocked reactivity to anger and fear in a face recognition task while enhancing happiness ratings if the participant experienced REM sleep. These research findings may help us further understand dreaming's role in people's lives and support a healing perspective regarding our nightly activities.

During dreamwork such as Embodied Imagination, much as in waking life, the human brain tends to scan for, recall, and react to unpleasant experiences. While this happens automatically, we can concurrently strive to embody and integrate positive, pleasing emotional experiences. This integration process may include holding the tension between two opposing sensory and emotional states, a dynamic that stimulates both the parasympathetic and autonomic nervous systems.

Neuropsychologist Rick Hanson compared this holding together of disparate emotional states to how mental activity creates new neural structures. He posited that much as one's body is built from the foods one eats, one's mind is constructed from the experiences one has. This construction may occur even while one is dreaming. Dream content shows a bias toward exhibiting unpleasant and alarming events over pleasant ones. Additionally, the emotions the dreamer experiences are more likely to be negative than positive. This highlights the idea that dreams may be hard to understand because they may unconsciously be disguised for various functional reasons. For example, a person may want to warn himself about danger while subconsciously needing to deny the danger. It is possible that by integrating particular experiences in an embodied way, dreamwork may help break the patterned cascade of trauma responses and behaviors that impede healing for those who have experienced trauma.

There is now sufficient research to support the idea that our physical health suffers as a result of stress and unprocessed emotional trauma. Neuroscientist and pharmacologist Candace Pert's research shows that a form of chemical communication through our cells happens in the body all of the time. She refers to this phenomenon of cellular chemical messengers as "the second brain," whereby the bloodstream, rather than the nervous system, carries select and important communication through the body. Pert believes that "unconscious emotions are stored in the body where they result in restricted blood flow." She claims that these withheld emotions are released and experienced in sleep and that making them conscious through dreamwork has a healing effect. During dreamwork, the individual experiences the emotional states found in dream images and realizes them through associations and embodiment, which can lead to integration and healing.

Many crises in people's lives have a long, unconscious history that they can integrate through dreams and a willingness and ability to attend to what dreams show them. Traumatic implosions set off in childhood can create profound relational and neurobiological cascades. As a result, the wounded individual's consciousness is often overwhelmed by archetypal content. However, once the individual comes into relationship with these archetypes, defenses can give way to psychological healing, growth, and increased creativity. This theory need not apply only to trauma suffered in childhood or to personality disorders, but to all types of trauma, as dreamwork can establish a healing relationship with the archetypes.

Once healers and patients alike embrace both the science and the spirit behind dreamwork, they will find that a holistic approach that includes guided dreamwork will ultimately result in more comprehensive treatment and greater potential healing than that without dreamwork. As psychologist and dream researcher Guy Dargert states, "if we cannot hear the message of the dream or the voice of the daimon in the dream we may find it necessary to respond to a more compelling manifestation of the image." Physical and psychological illnesses and their symptoms might manifest from the inner world just as much as from the outer world.

Ideally, in the near future, healers of all kinds can find a way to view symptoms as guideposts to those places that need our attention, places rich in the archetypal imagery associated with that which must be made conscious. Perhaps recent scientific insights into how the brain works in sleep and dreaming can help bridge the chasm between evidence-based medical practices and traditional and alternative practices. In the interest of healing, perhaps we can embrace the idea that just as your body is built from the foods you eat, your mind is built from the experiences you have, even while dreaming.

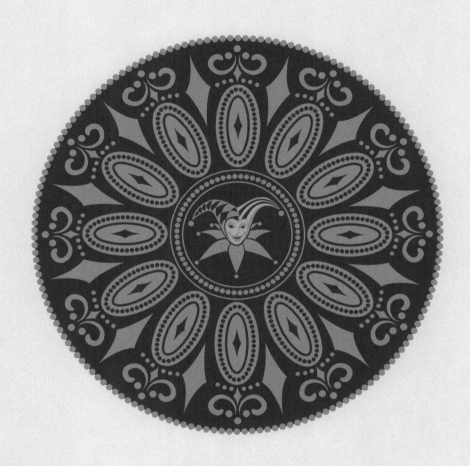

A GUIDED DREAM JOURNAL

- fini -

For more information on the neuroscience of dreaming, mysticism and dreaming, dreamwork for the dying, upcoming trainings and workshops and more please visit **www.DreamsHeal.com**

CPSIA information can be obtained
at www.ICGtesting.com
Printed in the USA
BVHW092338281221
625046BV00008B/722